The Must-Have User's Guide to

Treatments for Aging Skin

Elle Kersey

Editor

Marjorie Kramer

Disclaimer and Terms of Use

Effort has been made to ensure that the information in this book
is accurate and complete. However, the author and the
publisher do not warrant the accuracy of the information, text,
and graphics contained within the book due to the rapidly
changing nature of science, research, known and unknown facts,
and the internet. The author and the publisher do not hold any
responsibility for errors, omissions, or contrary interpretation of
the subject matter herein. This book is presented for
motivational and informational purposes only.

Dedication

This book is dedicated to all the women who did not have this information prior to making cosmetic choices that resulted in non-optimal results. Your challenges are what opened my eyes to the need for this book.

This book is dedicated to all the women who are in search of options that make them feel beautiful but does not negatively affect their health.

This book is dedicated to all my clients for the support, the love, the kindnesses, and willingness to share themselves and their issues with me.

This book is dedicated to my daughter for being wonderful, kind, understanding, and helpful on the front lines through all the ups and downs of my journey.

This book is dedicated to my family for being understanding when work has consumed me.

This book is dedicated to my father for being my rock my whole life.

Table of Contents

Introduction

The impetus to write this guide began before I even considered any of the information included here. In 1993, I gave birth to a beautiful baby girl. My pregnancy was complicated, and she was delivered by emergency caesarian section. To further complicate matters, my latex allergy caused me to have excessive internal scar tissue. If you have ever had surgery, you know that scarring is just part of what happens. Sometimes the scarring doesn't cause problems, but for me, there were major problems; so much so that I had to have several surgeries to remove scar tissue.

Scar tissue performs like an internal bandage. When it gets out of control in the abdomen, it can cause blockages of the intestines. This has happened to me multiple times. My surgeon tried many alternatives to figure out why I was having such an issue with this awful problem. During this insanity, my primary care physician moved away, and my new primary doctor said, "If you keep going like this, you are going to die." So after much conversation between my new primary doctor and my surgeon, the new protocols for latex allergies, and my understanding of what I could do to help myself, my last surgery was over ten years ago.

After doing much research on the subject of scar tissue, I realized that something I was familiar with was the best treatment for it. To my surprise, microcurrent is one of the best ways to address the reduction of scar tissue. As I started working on myself, I quickly realized that not only was the scar tissue getting better, but also my belly area was looking better and taking on a better shape. I began to share my discoveries with other women.

What I quickly comprehended was that scar tissue is rampant. Even if you don't get life-threatening blockages like mine, you can have real challenges that you don't even know are related to scar tissue. You can get scar tissue from having a baby, a car accident, urinary tract infections, and many more ways. It does not have to be a surgery or an open wound. Many of us try to work out and may do crunches for hours, and still not get the result that we want. It could be scar tissue that is preventing you from having the flat belly that you are looking for.

This realization led to my desire to create the highest standards of microcurrent usage to improve the human body. I created the QuadCore System, which utilizes microcurrent in the most profound way to improve the looks and function of the body.

My business, The Nonsurgical Aesthetic Institute, uses the QuadCore System to perform nonsurgical face and body lifts, scar therapy, cellulite therapy, rosacea, and acne treatments. QuadCore is offered as the healthy alternative in anti-aging treatments.

What I have found is that many women have not discovered the microcurrent option until they have tried other methods and/or have been found not to be candidates, are not happy with the results, or are at their wit's end with no relief. Other women have found microcurrent because they are looking for a healthy choice to the more well-known anti-aging options. Most people just want to look more refreshed but still look like themselves without the potential side effects associated with surgery. Hollywood has presented the best and worst of these options. Shocking outcomes like Priscilla Presley and Kenny Rogers are well documented in the press, but wonderful microcurrent faces like Jennifer Lopez and Princess Diana are not.

My mission is twofold. I want to move the conversation about anti-aging into a healthier direction, and I want to help women find anatomically harmonious options to reach a more youthful appearance. We have been told that the only way that we can look more youthful is to burn it out, cut it out, suck it out, or inject it in. I don't agree. I see it happen every day without any of that.

My opinion is simple; that surgery is for when you want to look anatomically different than you do naturally. Minimally invasive options are for tweaking certain portions of your anatomy, and microcurrent is for rejuvenating and re-energizing the tissue that you have.

I am slightly biased toward microcurrent because it made my life so much better, but I do know that every option has its place. It is your duty to find out which of them, if any, is the right one for you.

It is okay to take your time on this. You only get one body, and you have to live with whatever the ramifications are of the choices that you make. So be fully informed and choose wisely.

Elle

Avoid The Common Pitfalls

When you want to do something about your body's visual aging, educating yourself about all aspects and choices is paramount. Something as fundamental as getting a second opinion is overlooked way too often and can lead to unwanted results.

I wrote this guide to act as a beginning step when you are searching through the options in anti-aging. I believe that everything has its place in the beauty spectrum. The challenge is understanding and navigating the various options to reach the outcome you desire.

I have worked with thousands of women who have been in search of anti-aging help. The basic challenge is matching available options to your lifestyle and needs. Surgery requires time off from work. Injections are toxic and do not support a healthy lifestyle. Conversely, many of the "natural" options don't yield real results in a timely manner or can be difficult to implement.

So selecting options and products can get complicated if you don't understand the landscape. The goal is to help you understand, in real terms, the background of a product, what it is, how it affects the body, and what you can expect post-treatment.

It is not my mission to instruct you on what your choice should be, but rather to share information that can help you more easily identify the right selection for you.

As the beauty industry is an evolving entity, I invite you to join our Facebook Community as a resource for reliable information.

How To Use This Guide

This book is not designed to divert you from sound medical advice. This is a tool to help you have productive conversations with your physician during your selection process.

Medical professionals should take your needs, medical history, and special requirements into mind prior to any elective cosmetic procedure.

We are going to cover different kinds of treatments in groups as opposed to specific brand names. Brands change and new ones are always popping up. Broad strokes here can be drilled down and used for specific options that you find.

According to a quote from American Society of Plastic Surgeons website, www.plasticsurgery.org, Dr. Song asserts that selecting a Board Certified Physician is one of the most important choices in selecting your doctor.

Doctor Pre-Selection

The pre-work portion of the process is the most critical. This is where you find out all the professional credentials of your potential surgeon. Things you want to know are:

1. Are they board certified?
2. What is their patient mortality rate?
3. What kinds of reviews are online that are not related to the doctor's websites?
4. Does the doctor have privileges at local hospitals?
5. Are they currently being sued? Why?
6. Is the doctor currently under malpractice investigation?

This is just the starting point for doctor selection. You are putting your life in their hands. Every medical intervention is serious, and you cannot take it lightly. *Always get a variety of opinions from different doctors. Every procedure has nuances and differing ways for it to be done. The key is to find the procedure and process that is right for you.*

A routine procedure is only routine for the doctor. It is not routine for you and your body! The doctor can do everything that they are supposed to do, but your body, your health, your pre- and post-surgical exposures are the wild cards. Even though the doctor has taken every precaution, you can still have atypical or unusual results.

Some people keloid, some have hyper-adhesion production, some are slower to heal than others. There's also the level of stress in your life, unrealized pre-existing conditions, pets, chemical exposures, too much sun exposure.... The list of variables that can adversely affect the outcome of your procedure goes on and on.

Always ensure that you are selecting a professional, licensed, and certified physician.

Relevant Terminology

There are three main segments of surgery. Understanding the differentiation of these options allows you to weigh recovery time and the degree of body trauma to anticipate. For example, an **open surgery** is going to have more swelling and scarring than a minimally invasive procedure. Open surgery is surgery that requires an incision. These are considered the most invasive of all procedures. Open surgery should always be your last resort.

Minimally invasive procedures include a break in the skin or an entry into an orifice. Examples include injections, endoscopies, laparoscopies, catheterizations, and other procedures that are designed to have less downtime and create less damage to the body than traditional open surgical procedures. Minimally invasive procedures require less recovery time, but in some cases, they do not guarantee less pain or fewer side effects.

This option has become the fastest growing segment under the plastic surgery umbrella. The idea of quick fixes that get you in and out quickly, have lower costs, and have very little or no downtime seem to meet the needs of a growing number of people.

Noninvasive procedures do not break the skin and do not create direct contact to the internal body cavity.

This option fits more of a healthy lifestyle because it not toxic and requires no downtime. The biggest challenges with these kinds of services is selecting a skilled technician.

Anatomically harmonious procedures would be the most ideal because they would be noninvasive, nontoxic, have no recovery time, and show immediate improvement.

Post Procedure Preparations

When it comes to elective, cosmetic procedures, the more that you understand about what is going to happen during the procedure is just as important as knowing what the anticipated outcome will be.

Once you have identified the right procedure for you, the next step is to select the right person to take you through the procedure. When selecting a doctor, for example, they must be Board Certified and have experience in your exact procedure. Just because they are good at knees does not mean they will be good with eyes. The doctor or technician performing your procedure can make or break the outcome of a tried and proven procedure.

Do your research. Read reviews that are of an independent nature, not associated with the doctor. Request to speak with a client who has had your exact same procedure. Remember that skin type is important when reviewing past results. Are you prone to hyperpigmentation or scarring? Is your skin thin or prone to bruise easily?

There are no guarantees in surgical procedures because everything could go right in the operating room, but your health, the way that you heal, or an unexpected contact with something foreign after the procedure could cause an unanticipated result.

One last tip in this area. The body is the only thing that can heal the body. Actual meaningful rest is the best action that you can take to help get the result that you would like. Surgery is a trauma that requires proper rest and nutrition to recover from.

Prior to any procedure:

1. Ensure that correct emergency contact information is part of your chart.

2. Ensure that your emergency contact is aware of what you are doing and where.

3. You should always have someone be with you and care for you for a minimum of 24 hours after a procedure.

4. Be sure that you are fully aware of what your postsurgical situation will be and what the restrictions will be.

5. Always prepare for the worst reaction to a procedure and hope for the best.

6. Be patient with yourself. Healing varies from person to person. Take all the time you need to ensure that you have the best recovery possible.

7. Ensure that you know when and/or how to use the doctor's emergency number just in case you need the doctor's guidance in the early hours posttreatment.

8. Don't be embarrassed or afraid to ask questions or change your mind. If you feel that something is not right or you are having second thoughts, that is alright. You can always reschedule or skip the procedure all together.

Review of Popular Procedures

Botulinum Toxin Derivatives

Minimally invasive procedure

Top brands: Botox, Dysport, Myobloc, Xeomin

What is it?

Clostridium Botulinum is an anaerobic bacterium that produces the most toxic neurotoxin known to man. This bacterium can contaminate food and cause various degrees of sickness up to and including death.

Background

Though the original idea behind harvesting the toxin was to design a bioweapon during World War II, the ability to effectively and undetectably distribute the toxin to the enemy caused it not to be viable as a weapon. The technology was sold to Allergan and is now used for medical and cosmetic purposes.

How does it affect the body?

Neurotransmitters pass communication along the synapses of the body. Botulinum toxin derivatives disrupt the communication of these specialized cells and their offspring to cause a temporary disconnect of the brain and the body. This disconnect causes a paralysis of the targeted area.

What to expect

There can be issues like swelling, headaches, and bruising at the injection site. These issues vary from person to person and treatment to treatment. Avoiding blood thinners and alcohol prior to injections helps reduce these kinds of issues.

According to Wikipedia, the warning labels express this ideal this way:

In January 2009, the Canadian government warned that botulinum toxin products can have the adverse effect of spreading to other parts of the body, which could cause muscle weakness, swallowing difficulties, pneumonia, speech disorders, and breathing problems.

In April 2009, the FDA updated its mandatory box warning, cautioning that the effects of the botulinum toxin may spread from the area of injection to other areas of the body, causing symptoms similar to those of botulism, and that these adverse reactions, which were more likely in cases ignoring approved use guidance and label directions, could result in patient death.

Helpful Questions Prior to Injections

The successful mindset to have when considering these injections is that it is a serious undertaking. This is medication that will alter your body, and even though the delivery method is minimally invasive, the short- and long-term effects are not.

Prior to injections, you need to:

1. Discuss medications that you are already on. Drug interactions can be fatal.

2. Select only certified injectors that are verified by your manufacturer. This gives you a greater chance of getting clean product. Don't be afraid to ask to see the bottle the product came from. Black market and other products have been used to increase profits by some injectors in the past.

3. Ask which area of sites your injector specializes in. Make sure that you select someone who has experience in treating the area you want adjusted.

4. Always visit the website of your potential product and see what new information is available. Don't leave it up to your injector to be up on the latest information about your injectable.

Minimally invasive procedure

Top Brands: Juvederm, Restylane, Radiesse

What is it?

Fillers are made of various chemicals that are used to fill in unwanted hollows in the face. These are called "natural" because they are in a base that is "natural." However, in reality, they are chemical compounds that are manufactured and are not "natural" in the lay term.

Background

The first fillers were fat graphs used to improve cosmetic appearances in the 1800s. The first FDA-approved soft tissue augmentation product was in 1981. In 2003, the first hyaluronic acid-based products were FDA approved. In recent years, new products that address many issues associated with unwanted hollows of the face have been approved. Over the years, many varieties of fillers have also been approved.

How does it affect the body?

These types of products are supposed to pass through the body over time. This option is introduced into many aspects of the face like lips, cheeks, chins, under eyes, and in jawlines.

Understanding that there is a range of variety in composition means there is a range in the types of side effects. Therefore, understanding the chemical makeup of the type of injections and their typical side effects is critical.

What to expect?

1. Temporary relief of facial lines and greater fullness in the face.

2. Concerns at the time of injection: Swelling, bruising, rejection, and/or infection at injection site.

3. From day one to day seven, the level of result that you want should be realized.

Known potential side effects:

1. Hardening of the product in the skin, balling of the product under the skin, and migration of the product to other areas of the face.

2. Birth defects in unborn children.

3. Allergic reaction, cancer, pain, swelling and inflammation at the injection site.

It is important to ask your physician:

1. What product do they think is best for your specific issue?

2. What are the potential negative side effects associated with this drug?

3. What side effects, good or bad, have they observed firsthand?

4. How familiar are they with treating your specific concern?

5. Do they have "before and after" pictures of actual clients?

6. Ask specific questions about your second worst case scenario concern. (Worst case is death, so other than that.)

7. Ask what you should do if something unexpected happens, if 911 is not called. Inform your home care attendees of the answer to this question.

Top Procedures: laser hair removal, intense pulse light (IPL) or photo facial, skin resurfacing

Noninvasive procedure: Non-ablative laser does not damage the surface of the skin.

Minimally Invasive: Ablative laser procedures remove the outer layer of skin.

What is it?

The word "laser" is an acronym for *light amplification by stimulated emissions of radiation*. These kinds of procedures focus radiation into the body to destroy or interrupt the normal function of the tissue or its components to achieve the desired cosmetic result.

Background

The history of laser starts with the discovery of x-rays in 1895. By 1896, the concerns of the negative effects of radiation on the body began. Practical use of x-rays began in 1897 in hospitals during the Spanish-American War. Skip ahead to 1907, and reports were beginning that radiation was causing mutations in frogs. Then in 1911, a patient died from radiation injections. Findings linking x-rays with leukemia and cancer begin to appear. Not until 1931 do parameters for safer use come into being after years of various types of cancers being linked with overexposure. In 1947, the Atomic Bomb Casualty Commission was established to research the radiation poisoning associated with the atomic bomb on Japanese survivors of Hiroshima and Nagasaki. In 1955, reports of adverse effects of radiation from various areas around bomb testing sites started to be reported. In 1957, it was report by Karl Morgan to the United States Congress that there are no safe levels of radiation exposure. In 1970, a study was published to show that there was an increased risk of cancer in children if the mother was exposed during prenatal care. In the 1980s, there started to be some debate of previous findings of radiation on the body. In the late 1980s, the first instances of evidence of radiation cancer was reported when adults began experiencing tumors caused by overexposure to radiation. In 1990, a book entitled *Cancer from Low-Dose Exposure: An Independent Analysis* said that there were no safe levels of radiation exposure. Although regulatory agencies continued to debate the fine points, in 2000, industries like European airlines started to train staff on low-dose radiation exposure and protection. In 2003, the Health Physics reported that DNA can be altered with low-dose radiation.

Research is still being done. Various types of lasers and uses of radiation are being developed regularly.

How does it affect the body?

Laser send bursts of radiation to affect the chromosomes of the cells to either kill or damage them. This damage is healed at various rates in the body, so repeated treatments to the same area are needed to achieve the desired cosmetic result. The intended malfunction is semi-permanent to permanent, depending on the success of the treatment.

What to expect?

Non-ablative lasers treatments are mildly uncomfortable. The range of the feeling of the sting is anywhere from the snap of a small rubber band to a bee sting for each pulse. The discomfort is usually just for the moment of the pulse. Once the service is complete, the discomfort is over unless the surface of the skin has been damaged by having been accidentally burned. Ablative laser treatments require numbing compounds and pain medications posttreatment.

Important information to have prior to treatment.

For cosmetic laser use, there are various scales to determine the right settings for your treatment. The correct settings are designed to prevent burns to the surface of the skin, to allow the targeted cells to be affected properly, and to increase the level of success of your treatment. So filling out the intake forms as completely and truthfully as possible is a critical step in the success of your service.

When it comes to laser, the experience of the technician is critical. Many times, doctors do not perform basic laser treatments themselves. They hire technicians to do the job while the doctor oversees the process. A bad laser technician can hurt you and impede your progress. Ensure that your technician is experienced, not just the doctor they work for.

Important questions to ask

1. Will the doctor or a technician be performing your services? Get this answer in writing.

2. Ask what your settings are on each machine. Verify for yourself that you are within your range each time you visit. Your regular technician could be out for some reason, and you need to know your settings.

3. Ask what kind of laser they plan to use on you. Explore the most up-to-date info on the type and brand of laser they use. Is it the most current technology for what you want to achieve? Is there new information of side effects? Is there a better option for you in terms of effectiveness for your skin type? What kind of reputation

does your facility have independent of their website and literature?

4. Ask questions about the written instructions that you do not understand.

5. Ensure that you have the contact information for the posttreatment injury line of your selected facility. Your body may not show immediate signs of injury but later may develop deep welt burns that turn into deep brown or white spots. Follow the instructions of the facility to ensure that you get the help that you need.

Surgery

Invasive procedure

Top Cosmetic Procedures: facelift, neck lift, breast augmentation, tummy tuck

What is it?

Surgery covers a variety of procedures that remove portions of the body and/or introduce foreign objects into the body. It requires a breach of the body cavity and usually requires some kind of anesthesia and recovery time.

How it affects the body.

These kinds of procedures cause the internal aspects of the body to be exposed to external elements, medical instruments, and air. Manipulation of these organs is used to achieve the desired goal.

Surgery has various consequences that are usual, such as internal and external scarring. Inflammation and pain are also expected. Painkillers, anti-inflammatories, and/or antibiotics are dispensed post-surgery to address these concerns.

With surgery, there is always risk of death, infection, death of the skin at the incision site, and other complications that have been well-documented throughout the years. You can have the best surgeon in the world, and everything can go right, but the result can still be devastating. There is great risk in surgery, so it should always be your last resort. You should always take it very seriously. What is routine for a practice is not routine for your body. You must prepare and protect yourself before and after surgery. Your result is just as much your responsibility as your doctor's.

What to expect

You should expect to feel groggy post-surgery. You will wake up in post-op, and the nurses will be trying to interact with you. Once you are fully awake, you will be prepped to go home or to your hospital room. If you are going home, then you must have someone take you home. You will not be able to or allowed to drive yourself.

You will not remember what happened during the procedure, but you will feel the discomfort associated with it. It can take up to years to fully recover, but you are encouraged to resume normal activity anywhere from days to weeks once the procedure is complete.

What questions to ask

This is more important for this procedure than any other because the changes that occur are permanent and will require further surgery to correct if need be. You must understand fully and completely before you have any procedure done: THEY CAN NOT PUT BACK WHAT HAS BEEN REMOVED! So if you are not happy with the outcome, you may just have to live with it.

1. Is your potential surgeon an expert in the procedure that you are having? They might be great at tummy tucks but not have experience doing faces.

2. You want to see at least five "before and after" photos of people who have had similar pre-surgery concerns as you do.

3. Read reviews that are not generated by their website. It is critical that you find recent reviews by multiple patients. Your doctor may have been the best years ago, but he may not be the best now.

4. Make sure that the credentials of your surgeon include their patients' mortality rate.

5. Anesthesia is a very critical part of procedure. Ask as much as you can about who your anesthesiologist will be. Find out the same information as 1-4 for the anesthesiologist if you can.

Microcurrent

Anatomically harmonious procedure

Top procedures: facelift, neck lift, body re-contouring, scar reduction, post-surgical and post trauma treatments

What is it?

Microcurrent procedures utilize micro-electrical pulses to encourage the cells of the body to function normally. In doing so, the functions of the body begin to improve and function properly. This creates a dramatic and immediate effect in the appearance of the skin. This improvement reduces fine lines and wrinkles, inflammation, and scarring while leaving the skin looking more vibrant and toned.

Background

The earliest medical documentation of the use of microcurrent was by Jean Jallabert in Switzerland in 1749. Then in 1930, Carlo Metteucci documented electrical current in damaged tissue. Not much progress had been made in this field until 1969 when L. E. Wolcott and his team proved that using microcurrent on wounds hastened their healing rate. Then in 1991, Drs. Erwin Neher and Bert Sakman won the Nobel Prize for developing a way to detect the electrical currents of cell membranes. In the 1990's, microcurrent was approved for cosmetic purposes in Europe followed by the United States around 2009.

How does it affect the body?

The body has various frequencies that it uses to pass information throughout the body. When microcurrent is applied to the skin, it mirrors these frequencies to increase the ability of the affected area to remove and eliminate damaged cells or correct the activity levels or functions of subpar cellular activities.

What that looks like to the naked eye is faster healing of tissue, a more youthful appearance to the surface of the skin, and a more supple, softer feel of the skin. This is why it is ideal for an anti-aging treatment.

What to expect

Microcurrent for anti-aging has a variety of application options. It can range from unmanned adhesive electrodes to manned single wand technician handsets. Each provides a gentle influx of microcurrent into the skin that is painless and soothing. Depending on the application, it can feel like a massage or like nothing is happening. Once your time is up, you should be able to see a visible improvement in the treated area. There can be increased blood flow to the area, and a temporary redness can be evident. No recovery time or post-treatment is needed.

When it comes to microcurrent treatments, the skill of the technician and the techniques that they are trained to use will determine the level of results that are possible and how long those results will last.

What you should know

Microcurrent is not new, but the application for beauty has been neglected over the years. The various forms of its application have been developed by manufacturers to fit the various options in application.

Most technicians utilize the processes provided by manufacturers. Nonsurgical Aesthetic Institute is a leader in the advancement of the use of cosmetic microcurrent. We have created the QuadCore System, which is propelling the use of microcurrent to achieve full body enhancements.

The most important factors for a great outcome is the skill level of your technician and the techniques they use.

Helpful Questions

Have they used microcurrent in the area that you want treated?

How long has your technician been using microcurrent in the area that you want to have treated?

1. Check customer reviews on sites that are not provided by the facility.

2. Will a technician be present in the room during the entire treatment?

3. What kind of conducting agent do they use?

4. How often are treatments recommended?

Conclusion

Be prepared and empowered

What I suggest as an steadfast rule is, do your research! Just because something sounds good and your friend tried it does not suggest that it is going to be good for you.

There will always be the latest and the greatest. There will always be new technology, services, and information. Even though I did not go over it here, in my book, *Stop Wasting Money In The Skin Care Maze*, I do cover products in depth. That book is my next release.

In the beginning of this book, I spoke of joining our community. I write a blog called "Naked Gab." You can find it at www.nakedgab.com. We also have a Facebook page where you can give feedback on this book and ask related questions: https://www.facebook.com/mhugtfas. There are also printable worksheets available at: http://bit.ly/2rYOpal. These worksheets can help you prepare yourself for your journey into aging skin treatments and beyond. I hope this guide helps you avoid most of the novice pitfalls during your quest to look great at any age.

Elle

www.ingramcontent.com/pod-product-compliance
Lightning Source LLC
Chambersburg PA
CBHW061936280526
45787CB00004B/1627